CIRRHOSIS DIET

A guidebook on diet recipes to treat and prevent liver disease

Dr Rowan Theo

Table of Contents

CHAPTER ONE

What to Eat When You Have Cirrhosis

It's now no longer unusual for human beings with cirrhosis to emerge as malnourished because of adjustments of their metabolism and digestive troubles that arise because the liver turns into extra broken.

As such, when you have this circumstance, what you devour and drink every day is mainly vital, specifically as additives like protein, sodium, and sugar require your liver to paintings harder—a call for it is able to now no longer be capable of meet.

A cirrhosis diet regime ought to be crafted with the assist of your healthcare company and different individuals of your healthcare team, consisting of a registered dietitian, to make certain that you are competently nourished and fending off picks which can get worse your circumstance and in any other case effect your fitness.

Benefits

The liver has extra than 500 functions, making it one of the maximum essential organs.1 If your liver is broken from cirrhosis, it isn't capable of effectively carry out one in all its maximum vital tasks: supporting your frame get nutrients from the meals you devour.

A cirrhosis eating regimen can assist offer ok nutrients, lessen the quantity of labor your liver desires to do, thwart associated headaches, and save you in addition liver harm. Research has proven that human beings with liver sickness who are not competently nourished are much more likely to enjoy headaches from cirrhosis, together with death.

Liver Cirrhosis and Alcohol

How It Works

Your cirrhosis eating regimen will want to be tailor-made primarily based totally to your usual fitness and person desires, however there are a few trendy nutritional pointers that regularly form this ingesting plan:

• Avoiding alcohol: Any quantity is taken into consideration dangerous for every body with cirrhosis, as it is a ability motive of extra liver harm—even liver failure. Drinking also can make contributions to malnutrition and different fitness concerns.

• Limiting fat: The frame digests fat the use of bile, a yellow-

inexperienced fluid made in the liver. When the liver is broken, the manufacturing and deliver of bile can be affected, main to digestive signs. A liver that isn't running nicely has a tough time processing a excessive-fats meal. (Healthy fat may be blanketed in moderation.)

• Avoiding uncooked or undercooked meat/seafood: People with liver harm from cirrhosis have impaired immune function, which means micro organism and viruses that those ingredients can harbor can cause a doubtlessly severe infection.

In addition to converting the content material of your eating regimen, you could want to alternate the amount of the meals you devour. Having liver sickness can boom your chance for malnourishment, so that you can also additionally want to devour extra energy in an afternoon to fulfill the elevated electricity needs to your frame because of your circumstance.

If you've got liver sickness, realize that the suggestions for protein consumption vary. The have an impact on of protein on liver sickness is quite arguable and nonetheless being studied.6

You'll want to discuss with your healthcare company or a dietitian to decide the precise quantity of protein endorsed for you. The energy from protein can be an crucial factor of a numerous and nutritious eating regimen, and protein is fundamental to stopping muscle atrophy (thinning).

In a few cases, your healthcare company can also additionally need you to make extra, unique adjustments in your eating regimen to assist control or save you different situations human beings with liver cirrhosis can be much more likely to get.

CHAPTER TWO

Duration

If you're at chance for liver sickness, your healthcare company can also additionally need you to observe a cirrhosis eating regimen even in case you don't experience sick. Someone in the early tiers of liver sickness (compensated phase) commonly doesn't have any signs.

Signs of liver sickness can also additionally take years to reveal up, and that they achieve this most effective as soon as harm to the liver has emerge as severe (decompensated phase).eight

Since converting the way you devour can most effective assist save you extra liver harm, however can't heal what's already occurred, you'll possibly want to be on a cirrhosis eating regimen for a protracted time.

What to Eat

If you're following a cirrhosis eating regimen, there are a few ingredients and liquids you'll want to strictly keep away from. However, you'll have your preference of many nutritious and engaging ingredients, together with sparkling produce, entire grains, and plant-primarily based totally protein.

Compliant

• Fruits and vegetables (uncooked or cooked with out butter, oil, or salt)

• Eggs, egg whites

• Cooked fish (salmon, tuna)

• Lean hen or turkey (with out the skin)

• Low-fats Greek yogurt

• Cream cheese, ricotta

• Hard cheeses (cheddar, mozzarella)

• Nuts and seeds (unsalted)

- Dried beans and legumes

- Nut butters (unsalted)

- Tofu

- Fortified milk options (almond, soy, rice)

- Margarine

- Oats

- Whole grain bread, crackers, and cereals

- Brown rice

- Olive oil

- Fresh herbs

- Low-fats milk

- Garlic

• Ginger

• Quinoa, couscous

• Granola and cereal bars

• Coconut water

• Meal/dietary supplements, as permitted

Non-Compliant

• Raw or partly uncooked fish and shellfish (e.g., oysters, clams)

• Fast meals, fried meals

• Red meat

• Canned meals (meat, soup, vegetables)

• Packaged, processed snacks and food (incl. frozen)

• Hot dogs, sausage, lunchmeat

• Sauerkraut, pickles

• Buttermilk

• Tomato sauce or paste

• Instant warm cereal or oatmeal

• Potato chips, pretzels, rice cakes, crackers, popcorn

• Refined white flour pasta, bread, and white rice

• Oils excessive in trans fats or partly hydrogenated oils (palm oil, coconut oil)

• Breading, coating, and stuffing mixes

• Full-fats dairy merchandise

- Bread, biscuit, pancake, and baked proper mixes

- Pastries, cake, cookies, muffins, doughnuts

- American, Parmesan, Swiss, blue, feta, cottage cheese, cheese slices or spreads

- Pudding, custard, or frosting mixes

- Table salt, sea salt, blended seasonings

- Ketchup, soy sauce, salsa, salad dressing, steak sauce

- Bouillon cubes, broth, gravy, and stock

• Caffeinated tea, coffee, and gentle drinks

• Alcohol

Fruits and vegetables: Choose sparkling produce whilst possible, as canned types commonly have sodium and sugar. Add fruit to cereal or oats for additional nutrients, fiber, and a bit herbal sweetness. Fiber-wealthy culmination like apples make a wholesome and pleasant snack on their very own.

Dairy: Full-fats dairy merchandise will possibly be too tough in your frame to digest. Stick to low-fats Greek yogurt, small quantities of low-sodium tough cheese, and fortified dairy-unfastened milk options like almond or soy.

Rich, milk-primarily based totally cakes like pudding, custard, and ice cream ought to be limited. You can also additionally want to keep away from them absolutely on a cirrhosis eating regimen when you have tremendous problem processing fats and sugar.

Grains: Choose entire-grain bread, pasta, brown rice, and cereal in place of the ones made with delicate white flour. Granola and granola bars can be permitted for short snacks so long as they're low in sugar and sodium.

Protein: Red meat isn't permitted for a cirrhosis eating regimen, neither is any sort of processed lunch meat or sausage. Small servings of lean rooster with out the skin, a few kinds of sparkling-stuck fish (consisting of salmon), and eggs or egg whites can be suitable.

The majority of your protein allowance ought to come from plant-primarily based totally reassets consisting of dried beans and legumes, small quantities of unsalted nuts or nut butter, and tofu.

Desserts: Packaged cake, cookie, brownie, biscuit, pancake, and waffle mixes may be excessive in sugar and salt, so it is quality to keep away from them. In trendy, you'll need to keep away from pastries, doughnuts, and muffins, except you could make your very own low-fats, low-sugar, and low-salt versions.

Beverages: You can not drink alcohol when you have liver cirrhosis, however you may have masses of different alternatives. Water is the maximum hydrating preference, however in case you are on a low-sodium eating regimen, you'll need to test the labels on bottled water as a few comprise sodium. Milk and juice ought to most effective be ate up if pasteurized.

While a few studies has advised coffee (however now no longer different caffeine-containing liquids) may want to have advantages for human beings with liver sickness because of alcohol use, maximum clinical experts suggest that sufferers with cirrhosis keep away from caffeinated liquids, together with coffee, tea, and gentle drinks.

CHAPTER THREE

Does Coffee Prevent Liver Disease?
Recommended Timing

Liver sickness can cause malnourishment, wherein case your healthcare company may need you to devour extra energy. If you don't experience as much as ingesting large food to boom your caloric consumption, strive ingesting small, common food and snacks during the day.

Some human beings with liver sickness locate they awaken in the night time. They can also additionally live wakeful for lengthy stretches and turn out to be taking naps at some point of the day. If you're wakeful in the center of the night time, studies has proven that having a late-night time snack (mainly the ones which have been particularly formulated for this purpose) may be useful for human beings with cirrhosis.

If your sleep agenda is interrupted, make sure that you're making plans your food round while you are wakeful, whether or not it's at some point of the day or at night time. Try now no longer to head longer than more than one hours with out a meal or snack.

Cooking Tips

Try grilling or boiling greens and making ready them with out oil or butter.

If you're lowering your sodium consumption as a part of a cirrhosis eating regimen, strive the use of sparkling herbs and spices in place of desk salt.12If you're used to including salt in your meals and locate it tough to interrupt the habit, your healthcare company can also additionally will let you use a salt substitute.

When cooking meat, begin via way of means of deciding on lean cuts.

Skinless rooster is a more healthy alternative than beef.

You can be allowed to have small quantities of pork now and again relying on how it's prepared. For example, grilling meat in place of frying with oil or butter reduces the fats content material and stops it from turning into too greasy for a cirrhosis eating regimen.

In addition to fending off uncooked or partly cooked meat and seafood, exercise right meals coping with and protection practices to in addition lessen your chance of foodborne infections.

Modifications

You can also additionally want to conform your eating regimen in case you expand headaches from cirrhosis, consisting of ascites, hypoglycemia, and encephalopathy. If you expand one or extra of those situations, your healthcare company can also additionally advocate extra adjustments in your eating regimen, together with proscribing salt, sugar, and protein.

Ascites

Ascites is the buildup of huge quantities of fluid in the abdomen. Healthcare vendors commonly require a strict no-salt eating regimen for human beings who've cirrhosis with ascites, as sodium could make the circumstance worse.

Prepackaged and comfort meals gadgets are regularly excessive in sodium or comprise introduced salt. If you are now no longer mechanically checking the nutrients labels, you could now no longer be aware about how a good deal sodium you're consuming.

When you're doing all your grocery shopping, a very good rule of thumb is to recognition on what you could purchase alongside the fringe of the keep—sparkling produce, lean meats, and low-fats dairy—which can be low-sodium picks. Avoid the packaged snacks, cereals, and sodas determined in the center aisles.

Encephalopathy

As the frame digests protein, it creates a byproduct referred to as ammonia. When the liver is functioning nicely, that is cleared with out issue. But a broken liver cannot deal with a everyday quantity of protein, not to mention any extra.

The extra protein it attempts to digest, the extra ammonia can construct up. At excessive levels, it turns into poisonous to the mind and may motive reminiscence problems, dementia-like signs, and a severe hardship referred to as encephalopathy.

If you've got cirrhosis, recognition on together with plant-primarily based totally protein reassets for your eating regimen in place of meat. Your healthcare company can also additionally come up with a particular restriction of the way a good deal protein you could have according to meal or according to day.

Liver Disease and Hepatic Encephalopathy

CHAPTER FOUR

Hypoglycemia

Hypoglycemia, or low blood sugar, is some other common trouble if you have cirrhosis. When your liver is wholesome it shops electricity from the complicated carbohydrates you devour in an without difficulty available shape referred to as glycogen.

If you've got cirrhosis, your liver isn't capable of keep sufficient electricity on this chemical shape. As a result, human beings with liver sickness can also additionally enjoy episodes of low blood sugar.

Research has proven that ingesting excessive-fiber food with a low glycemic index can assist control hypoglycemia in human beings with cirrhosis.

An Overview of Hypoglycemia

Considerations

Since it's so vital to stay with your cirrhosis eating regimen, preserve the subsequent in thoughts to set your self up for success.

General Nutrition

Since you'll have your preference of sparkling culmination and greens, entire grains, and plant-primarily based totally reassets of protein, a cirrhosis eating regimen may be a nutritious one.

However, a few human beings who've liver sickness enjoy gastrointestinal signs consisting of nausea and lack of urge for food that make it tough for them to devour sufficient to live nicely nourished. In such cases, your healthcare company can also additionally have you are taking nutrients or dietary supplements.

Safety

Be cautious of dietary supplements or multivitamins that comprise a whole lot of diet A, which may be poisonous to the liver.17 You may also need to test together along with your healthcare company earlier than beginning any dietary supplements containing iron, which may be tough for the liver to procedure in excessive doses.

Approach natural or nutritional supplements advertised to "guide liver fitness" with caution. These dietary supplements could have aspect results in their very own, together with inflicting digestive signs or making them worse. And they could engage with medicinal drugs you've got been prescribed, the results of which may be severe.

Speak together along with your healthcare company earlier than attempting any of those merchandise.

Flexibility

Fat, sugar, and salt make for short and what many human beings consider "crowd-pleasing" ingredients. As such, they're regularly staples in food you get whilst eating out, making menus tough to navigate at the same time as on a cirrhosis eating regimen. Even what looks as if a compliant meal can also additionally percent extra punch than you think, given its element size.

Preparing your food at domestic is possibly quality.

Keeping an eye fixed out for hidden elements is likewise vital on the grocery keep. When you're shopping, don't forget that merchandise labeled "low-sodium" can be low in salt, however regularly have a whole lot of introduced sugar. If you're additionally lowering your sugar consumption on a cirrhosis eating regimen, those alternatives won't be suitable.

Dietary Restrictions

If you've got different nutritional desires and alternatives your healthcare company, in addition to a registered dietitian or nutritionist, allow you to regulate a cirrhosis diet regime to suit your desires.

For example, when you have celiac disease and can not have wheat or gluten, you'll need to cautiously pick out gluten-free bread, pasta, and crackers. Pasta options crafted from beans and legumes may be nutritious however can be too excessive in protein for a cirrhosis eating regimen.

If you already observe a plant-primarily based totally eating regimen, you won't ought to issue in lowering your beef consumption or fear approximately fending off sure kinds of shellfish. However, you could want to regulate your protein consumption in case you usually devour a eating regimen with masses of nuts and seeds or tofu.

THE END